Acknowledgment

There is really only one person I need to acknowledge for helping me write this book. Jamie Dant has been an amazing source of information, part-time editor, full time common sense checker, and the best wife a guy could have.

Thank you for introducing me to this diet and for putting up with my zany ideas about what I can do with it.

About the authors

Bronson Dant is the owner of Ellicott City Health and Fitness in Ellicott City, MD. He has spent several years helping people improve their health and fitness. Bronson has several levels of training and certifications in health and fitness. He is 46 years old and is also an active spokesperson for helping people over 40 stay young and on top of their game.

Jamie Dant is an owner of Ellicott City Health and Fitness and Outside the Box Nutrition. Her mission is to help people live healthy through education, habit building, and expert support. She has a Master's Degree in Integrative Health and Nutrition, and is a Board Certified and Licensed Nutritionist in the State of MD.

What you should know

Dr. Paul Mabry is a very vocal proponent of the Carnivore Diet (a.k.a. Zero Carb or ZC). With his permission I've included some excerpts of things he has written or said about this way of eating.

From Dr. Mabry's website http://borntoeatmeat.com

"One of the most common questions I get about low carb, high fat diets (LCHF) of all types, not just Zero Carb is "Isn't this going to cause me to have a Heart Attack". The answer is an emphatic "no", in fact, just the opposite is true. LCHF diets are the best way to avoid a heart attack. Yes, your total and LDL Cholesterol is likely to rise but these markers have nothing to do with heart attacks. The important tests found on a Cholesterol Panel that suggest you're in trouble are a Low HDL Cholesterol, a high serum Triglycerides and elevated levels of small, dense LDL Cholesterol particles. You need an NMR Cholesterol panel to measure the amount of small dense LDL Particles which most doctors rarely do. Eating LCHF will make all these risk markers as well another significant risker mark C-Reactive Protein (CRP) which measures inflammation go well into the green zone. Cholesterol is an innocent bystander in the crime of heart disease."

As Dr. Mabry points out, eating meat won't give you heart disease. In fact, many things you'll learn in this book run counter too much of what we've been taught about nutrition and how our bodies work.

From an interview he did on the Zero Carb Zen Blog.
https://zerocarbzen.com/2016/05/24/zero-carb-interview-dr-paul-mabry-m-d/

"One thing I've learned in my life is that consistency and discipline are the keys to success. I didn't get to be a "Full Bird" Colonel in the Army without them. If you fall off the wagon, get right back on, don't give up. Keep your eye on the goal. Hang a dress or pair of jeans you'd like to get back into where you'll see it several times daily. Hang out with people on Facebook who are having success with ZC like you and me."

Dr. Mabry hits on a critical idea. For most of you reading this book, cutting ALL carbs will be very difficult. You will probably fail more than once.

Keep at it. The only failure is giving up.

Find someone that can guide you. Associate with other people going through and dealing with the same things you are.

How does it work?

"Eat meat, Drink water", is the mantra of the carnivore community. The Carnivore Diet aka. The Zero Carb Diet has been an effective tool for many years to help people with all sorts of issues heal themselves and live better lives.

There is a long list of diseases, chronic illness, and other health factors that moving to an all meat diet has helped people improve and heal from.

Question: How does the Carnivore Diet do all this and help you lose body fat, gain muscle, and make you feel more energized?

Answer: Addition by subtraction

Some things we know.
1. Carbohydrates are used for fuel before body fat is used for fuel. As long as we have excess carbs in our systems, we'll never lose body fat.
2. Plant-based foods are basically carbs. Think about that for a minute…. Now think about number 1 on this list.
3. Fat provides more energy per gram (9 calories) than carbs do (4 calories). So fewer equals more. You have to eat more than 2 x the carbs to get the same amount of fuel.
4. Plant-based foods take an extraordinary amount of work to be broken down into anything useful. Most of the processes our bodies have to go through in order to digest and use nutrients we get from

plant-based food is multiples of what happens with meat. This is called bio availability.

5. Also, the by-products of all this extra work increase our dependence on more plant-based food and then additional processes needed to deal with the by-products and waste. Take a look at Vitamin C or fiber as an example.
6. One of the biggest issues facing our society is the rise in chronic inflammation. This condition presents in so many ways, it's almost pointless to list them all here.
7. The other major health issue we're dealing with is insulin resistance and the affect carbs have on managing Type 1 diabetes and creating Type 2 diabetes in more and more people every year.
8. Fat is not bad for you. You need it for almost every function of your body.

Addition by subtraction

The first thing the Carnivore diet does is get rid of all the carbs. This does a few things.

1. It allows the body to start burning body fat for fuel.
2. It eliminates the extra processing energy and bodily functions being used to get nutrients from plant matter
3. It eliminates the need for many currently thought to be "essential" supplements and compounds. Again, less extra stuff our bodies need to deal with.
4. It removes all factors that can adversely affect insulin resistance
5. It significantly reduces inflammation.

Just with that list of things the Carnivore Diet brings to the table, I often wonder why everyone isn't doing it already. The number of things that we deal with on a day to day basis that are a result of the things that carbohydrates do to our bodies is mind boggling.

It gets better.

With the Carnivore diet we get to lose fat, improve overall bodily function, and help our bodies heal over time. Here's how

1. The most bio available foods are meats. Also, the most highly nutrient food too. Less eating more nutrients
2. More fat. This is such a huge benefit of the diet. 60%-70% of the food you eat will be fats. You'll feel more full, have more energy, and your body will start to feel fresh again with more fat in your life.
3. Digestion issues usually go away. Again, less food, less waste. Less need for extra stuff to digest the food equals less digestion issues.
4. Easier to regulate gains and losses. Smaller changes in how much you eat can have a greater effect on the progress you make towards your goal.
5. No need for tons of supplements. It's all in the meat. Outside of a couple that we suggest everyone take no matter what diet you use, extra vitamins, minerals, powders, shakes, etc, ... can all go away.

In general, the Carnivore diet takes away the seriously bad stuff and replaces it with seriously good stuff. Your body will function better with less inflammation, less stress, and more energy available to fuel your active lifestyle.

Keep reading to find out more and how you can make this diet work for you.

Table of Contents

My Story

I wrote this as a blog post for our gym a while ago. It's kind of amazing how prophetic these words were. Everything you read in my story has led me to the Carnivore Diet. If you've followed my blog themeatlife.com then you know how I've progressed and how this story is evolving.

It doesn't take much to be extraordinary. Just be open the change and accept it into your life. Take this message with you as you read the rest of The Meat Life. I know you can make this work. If I can, it's can't be that hard.

It doesn't take much to be extraordinary

A few years ago I was 40 pounds overweight, and a sloppy mess. I went to the gym 3-4 times a week, but didn't really follow a plan, or put that much work into it.

I was going to the gym because it made me feel better about how poorly I was taking care of my body, not because I actually wanted to change anything about it.

I was in my late 30s, weighed 230 pounds on a good day, and I was holding on to about 25% body fat. My waist was +36 in., with disc herniations and pain in my neck, I slept horribly. My stomach issues were legendary.

Then one day it happened. My daughter took a picture of me at the beach one summer....

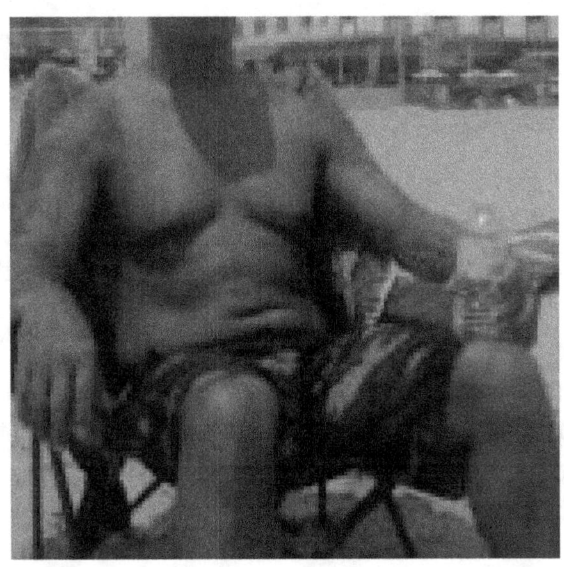

I had man-boobs!! My belly hung over my bathing suit and onto my lap! I had belly rolls! I was mortified. Was this really me? Yes, it was.

It was time to face the fact that I had let myself go. I didn't know then that the way I saw myself was nothing compared to where my health was. I hadn't made the connection between how I looked and how healthy I was. My initial reaction was solely based on my appearance.

Fast forward a few years…

I'm 45 years old. I weigh 195 pounds. I'm at 17% body fat. I wear 32in. pants now. I sleep like a rock. I still have disc herniations, but they don't bother me anymore. All my stomach issues have left me and the rest of the world is safe from harm. I still only workout 3-4 days a week. I'm stronger, more active, and can do more things than many people half my age.

How did I do it? How did I change from being overweight, unmotivated, and ignorant about health?

I did it one step at a time.

Looking at people that are living a "healthy" lifestyle, we get overwhelmed by all the things we see that are different than the way we are living our lives.

We see the regular exercise, the food prep, and healthy food choices, the reading and discussion of health topics, all the other healthy people they associate with….and we wonder how in the world they do it.

We think to ourselves, "I can barely get myself through a day right now, how can I add in an exercise program?". We say, "There is no way I could eat the way they eat, it must be horrible. Who has time to do all that work just to "be healthy?".

I was the same way, but I got lucky. I met people that helped me learn that if you focus on being healthy first, the way your body looks will follow along. I learned that if I change my mindset from trying to look good, to trying to perform better, my life would be forever changed.

I stopped looking at all the things I needed to change and focused on one change at a time.

This was easy because at first I didn't want to change a lot. I liked my french fries, and my morning Boston Cream donuts. I was only able to handle one small change at a time.

I learned how to exercise first. I joined a CrossFit gym and had coaches who trained me how to move my body, and follow an exercise program that made me work harder than I had been working, to see changes.

Then I started cutting back on fast food. This was the hardest. I learned how to prep my food for the week, and ate better during the day and saved some money too.

There are a lot of little things that I could talk about. The bottom line is that nothing happened overnight. Gradual changes happened as I'm ready for them.

The changes I've made, slowly over the last several years have helped me go from being an unhealthy slob to learning and studying fitness, to opening Ellicott City Health and Fitness.

My goal is to help educate people and help them make the first small step towards making the same changes I've made to improve their lifestyle and enjoy life better.

Being extraordinary just takes one small change. You can be extraordinary by taking one small step to own your fitness, change your level of performance day to day. You will feel better, look better, and be happier.

Chapter 1 - Why I wrote this book

A while ago my wife, Jamie, came to me with a half-cocked idea that I should try this thing she heard about called The Carnivore Diet. I asked her what it was, and she said it was just eating meat and nothing else.

Yeah right, ...

She was half joking but there was also a little bit of a serious tone in her suggestion that caught my attention.

You see Jamie is a certified and licensed nutritionist. She has been trying to get me to eat better for 10 years. She has succeeded in major ways, however, my system has always been, let's say "sensitive" when I consume too many vegetables. She's wanted me to go on an elimination diet for a while. I think this idea was her way of faking me into one.

I took her suggestion and put it aside for a couple weeks but it wouldn't leave me alone. I found myself looking it up and searching for information about it. I found some good blogs by people that have done it and started thinking that maybe this was something I wanted to try.

A little more about me.

I'm 46 years old. I own a gym, I coach CrossFit classes, I do personal training, and workout 3-5 days a week. I'm 6' tall and I weighed around 200 lbs when I started the Carnivore Diet. I was fairly healthy and there wasn't a real health reason (other than my previously noted "sensitivity" to too many veggies) for me to do this crazy diet.

As I learned more, I became intrigued about a few things.

I was tired of the seesaw of having to gain weight to get strong, then lose strength to get lean. From what others had experienced, I could potentially increase my strength and performance without gaining weight from fat. This has been something I have struggled with for years. Conventional wisdom says that in order to gain muscle you must have a higher carb intake. Do a Google search for "more carbs for more muscle" you'll see what I mean.

I'm lazy. One of the hardest things my wife has struggled with in her crusade to save my diet, has been my lack of interest in cooking. I'm a good cook. I just don't enjoy it. I'm the guy who will eat a can of tuna with some mayo before cooking the steak that's been sitting in the fridge. This diet looked simple, yet I would be eating things I'd never really taken the time to try.

There was something about the carnivore diet that rang true to me. The information and insights I picked up from people a lot smarter than me, were making me rethink what I thought I knew. This was a little intoxicating. I felt like I was learning something secret that only a few people knew. Maybe, if I could get into this club, I could use my information to change the broader view of people around me.

After a couple of weeks I saw a carnivore meme that was making fun of vegans and it got me thinking. I won't post the meme here because that's not what this book is about. I will say that the crux of the meme was that herbivore's eyes are on the side of their heads and carnivore's eyes are in front. This isn't breaking news. For me, something clicked. My brain went off into a million directions looking for more correlations to that idea.

How are carnivores different from herbivores and what traits do humans have that are similar? I'll save that general discussion for another time, but as you go through this book, remember that herbivores are designed to process plant matter. Then ask yourself, "If we were meant to be primarily plant eaters, why do we react to plant-based food the way we do?".

The beginning

When I started the Carnivore Diet I had no idea how to start what I was doing. For the first 12 days I ate eggs, bacon, Bulletproof coffee, hamburgers, salmon and top sirloin steak.

From there I looked for clues on how to do this the right way. I wanted to make sure I was getting the right nutrients, minerals and everything my body needed.

I learned about the importance of organ meat. I learned about several issues that aren't issues and a few things that are being used as guidelines that I think are wrong.

I quickly realized there had to be a better way to do the Carnivore Diet without making it up as I went.

I couldn't find one.

I found a dozen blogs of personal stories and anecdotes about what this person or that person has done. I found a chat group on WhatsApp with Carnivore dieters from all over the world who all had different recommendations to give me. There is a Facebook group with over 10,000 people in it that all have different opinions and ideas about what the diet means to them.

I was able to glean information from podcasts and make assumptions about various pieces of the puzzle from doing a lot of reading listening and information pruning.

In the absence of a single, helpful resource to point a potential carnivore in the right direction, I give you "All the meats".

What this book is

This book is simply my attempt at compiling into a single location, as much information as possible to help someone get started on the carnivore diet safely and enjoyably.

I am not a scientist, I cannot attest to anything specific about what the Carnivore Diet will do to you or anyone. I can only use my experience and what others have shared of theirs to provide a road map to help get someone started.

The information in this book has not been studied or tested outside the realm of "anecdotal evidence". If you try something and you have a different result please let the world know. The more information we have on this, the better we will all be.

If you use the information in this book to start the Carnivore Diet, all the results, reactions and effects on your body, mind and soul are on you.

If you are interested in the Carnivore Diet, I hope this book gives you a good base of knowledge to get started. I tried very hard to keep things simple, yet thoroughly explain things, so they made sense. If you are looking for more detailed explanations and hard data, there is a reference list at the end of the book with some fantastic resources for you to look into.

Esmée's Story

Esmée La Fleur, has been following the Carnivore Diet for a long time. With her permission, this is an excerpt of her story from her blog at zerocarbzen.com.

She started eating vegan at the age of 16 and tried several diets along the way. She has a great story of exploration and healing. She has tried fasting, a yogurt diet, fruitarianism, keto, raw meat and leafy greens, and eventually she found the Zero Carb a.k.a. The Carnivore Diet.

It's a good story make sure to check it out.
https://zerocarbzen.com/about-me/

She is a great example of being self-aware and trying different things until she found something that worked for her. The Carnivore Diet isn't something that has strict rules that must be followed. We are all individuals and if the common thoughts around what the diet is don't fit your lifestyle or needs, then it's OK to adjust to what's best for you.

"...I made the decision to follow the advice of Amber and several other long-term zero carb-ers to eat only meat and drink only water for 30 days. Essentially, it is the Zen version of the Paleolithic diet! By eliminating all other variables, it creates a clear baseline for comparison if you should decide to reintroduce dairy back into your diet. Most of those who have been practicing zero carb eating for a significant length of time say they feel best on a diet of only meat and water. Within a mere three days of making this

decision, I knew there was no going back. This is not just a diet; it is a way of life.

Since I discovered the Facebook group Zeroing In On Health, founded by several long-term zero carb-ers, I have met numerous individuals who have been living entirely on meat and water for anywhere from 5 -18 years, and have even given birth to and raised children on this diet. You can read about Kelly's personal journey on her blog My Zero Carb Life. Clearly, the importance of fruits and vegetables and even fiber in the diet has been highly overrated. In fact, according to Dr. Georgia Ede, MEAT contains ALL of the nutrients that humans need for optimal well-being. This makes perfect sense when you remember that a diet of only meat and water is, after all, the Original Human Diet.

It has been a long and interesting journey, but it sure is nice to finally be home."

Esmée is also involved in moderating a Carnivore focused group on Facebook called Principia Carnivora. Check it out. https://www.facebook.com/groups/PrincipiaCarnivora

Chapter 2 - What is the Carnivore Diet?

The simplicity of it all

It's simple, eat meat, drink water.

There are several explanations of why the Carnivore Diet makes sense. Some of them are based in theory some of them make sense scientifically. I'm not going to dive to far down those rabbit holes in this book. I'm assuming that you've already decided or are close to deciding to try the Carnivore Diet and have already looked into why you want to do it.

The main supporting ideas for the Carnivore Diet are:

The history of humans

Theories abound as to what ancient civilizations diets looked like. Many people claim that early man, (cavemen in the Paleolithic era), ate meat and nuts with little grain. Some say that meat was the primary source of food for millions of years. There are supporters of the vegan diet who claim that ancient Egyptians were vegetarians for 4000 years.

Personally, who cares?

My belief is that whatever happened hundreds, thousand, or millions of years ago doesn't have any bearing on the evidence, effectiveness, or value of the Carnivore Diet as we see it today.

What I've personally, experienced far outweighs what anyone could extrapolate from hypothetical research about cavemen.

Physiology and biology of humans

We have more in common with carnivorous animals than herbivorous animals. Our digestive tracts and our role at the top of the food chain, by definition, lends itself to eating meat as the primary source for fuel.

Scientific proof

Regardless of what we were told for most of our lives, fat is good, carbs are bad. There are dozens of studies that have been done over the years that show conclusively that fat is good for us. The information that is available debunking the correlation between low fat diets and heart disease is astounding. As a health and fitness professional this really gets me excited. This diet could (and does) drastically change people's lives. (See, Ref 15, 16, 17, 18)

It's an idea

Currently there is no governing body or committee that has convened to define the structure and operational parameters of what is considered The Carnivore Diet. There are a few people out there who are carrying the torch for the diet and have developed a following that has loosely developed some guidelines around the idea of the diet.

The basics are to eat only animal products and drink water. Of course everyone has their own goals and reasons for being on the diet so variations of the theme branch out from there.

Some people consider dairy to be OK on the diet others don't. Some say eggs are OK, others don't.

You'll find some people using sauces and some condiments, others won't.

I drink coffee every day, some would say I'm not doing the diet "correctly"

See where this is going??

My definition of the Carnivore Diet

The Carnivore Diet is a diet consisting primarily of animal meat products and by-products with the intention to supply the full range of nutrients and fat the body needs within the framework of a person's lifestyle.

Yup it's kinda open to interpretation and that's exactly how it should be.

No diet with an exacting protocol is going to do the same thing for everyone. People respond to things differently and any nutrition program should make variances for that.

A couple of things to keep in mind. The general goal of the Carnivore diet is to 1. Reduce carbohydrates, and 2. Significantly increase fat intake. Fat is good, eat all the fats, (naturally occurring fats of course).

Food quality is ALWAYS important. Many people that are doing the Carnivore diet aren't putting a lot of focus on the quality of what they are eating. You will see results either way, but if health is your goal, more than just losing body fat….go organic, grass fed, pasture raised, etc...

We're going to get into the most common guidelines you'll find on what is in or out of the Carnivore Diet. This is not comprehensive and you may find someone that disagrees with it. That's cool, it's not their list.

Eat it all

Meat	Dairy	Other Stuff
Beef	Full fat milk	Eggs
Fowl	Cheese	Ghee
Seafood		Bone Broth
Bison		Bone Marrow
Goat		Mustard
Lamb		No sugar seasonings
Pork		
Organ Meat		

Keep it away

Bread
Sugar
Vegetables
Nuts
Beans
Most Condiments

Somewhere in-between

Coffee

As you can see, it's pretty straightforward. If it walked or crawled you can eat it or something made from its body.

We won't get into food preparation and recipes in this book. I don't have that kind of time. If you aren't sure about something, think about why you're on the diet and how that thing will affect the result you're looking for. Think through the decision and you'll be fine.

Besides, if it doesn't work then learn from it and do it differently next time. There is no real way to get this wrong if you approach it as a learning experience.

How much do you need to eat?

The amount of food you eat is based on what your goals are. This is one thing that I have to disagree with most of what I've seen from people on the diet.

The most common advice you're going to get is Intermittent Fasting with 2 meals at about 2 pounds of meat each day.

You may also see the advice of eat until your full then eat again when you're hungry. I did this and in the first 12 days I lost 7 pounds. That's too much too fast. I figured out I was in an average 400 calorie deficit to my BMR (Base metabolic rate).

Neither of these are necessarily wrong, they just aren't right for everyone.

First define what your goals for the diet are. Do you want to lose body fat, gain muscle mass, reduce inflammation and joint pain, balance out your insulin spikes, or something else…?

This will help you with both amount and timing your meals. Remember, you're going to have to play around with it until you find what works best for you.

Because you are eating much more fat than you're used to, you will most likely feel full for longer periods of time and by default may eat less overall. You may need to force yourself to eat more at first until you get used to it.

The most important part of knowing how much to eat is tracking your meals, amounts, and what changes you see in yourself over time. Without data, you won't have any idea what's working or what you need to change to make it better.

My suggestion is to start by trying to eat at least enough calories to match your BMR. If you don't have access to any body composition technology, (InBody Scanner, or Bod Pod), you can find BMR calculators all over the Internet.

When I targeted my total calorie intake to at least meet my BMR, I lost weight, maintained muscle and lost fat.

Chapter 3 - Are you crazy?

The first few times you tell someone that you're just eating animal products and nothing else, you're going to get some blank stares, ... right before they unload a million questions and statements about how unhealthy and crazy you are.

Guess what you are a little crazy. So am I. We're doing this diet because it makes sense to us even though there isn't a lot of data to prove to us that it's not going to kill us. We're taking a leap of faith.

This is how the way people eat, especially with "fringe" diets, gets emotionally drawn into and starts to connect with how they identify themselves. Through this whole process remember that what you eat does not determine who you are. Don't take anyone's questioning or criticism of your choices personally.

Let's go through some of the most popular declarations of insanity.

You're going to get scurvy

Scurvy is a disease resulting from a lack of Vitamin C (ascorbic acid). Early symptoms include weakness, feeling tired, and sore arms and legs. Without treatment, decreased red blood cells, gum disease, changes to hair, and bleeding from the skin may occur. As scurvy worsens there can be poor wound healing, personality changes, and finally death from infection or bleeding (ref. 1)

Scurvy is the manifestation of a lack of collagen in the body. Collagen is the building block for our skin and other connective tissues. Basically if you don't get enough Vitamin C, you're going to die. Or will you?

What this reference doesn't tell you, nor do most of the references to scurvy, is that we only need vitamin C if we are eating plant based foods.

Vitamin C is required to convert the amino acids proline and lysine into hydroxyproline and hydroxylysine so that collagen can be formed in the body. In plant based foods proline and lysine are available but in their pre-hydroxylated form. Vitamin C is what brings them together.

Meat and animal products have hydroxyproline and hydroxylysine in them already. There is no need for Vitamin C because it wouldn't have anything to do in your system.

Vitamin C is required to form collagen in the body, and it does this – despite being described everywhere as an antioxidant – by oxidation. Vitamin C's role in collagen formation is to transfer a hydroxyl group to the amino acids lysine and proline. Meat, however, already contains appreciable quantities of hydroxylysine and hydroxyproline, bypassing some of the requirement for vitamin C. In other words, your vitamin C requirement is dependent upon how much meat you do not eat. (ref. 2)

Also, Glucose (carbs) take a higher processing priority in our body than Vitamin C. They use the same mechanism to get broken down for use. This is one of the reasons you need more vitamin C in your body if you are eating carbs. Your body doesn't process a majority of the vitamin C in what you eat because the carbs are taking all the seats on the train.

So basically 1. We don't need vitamin C if we don't eat carbs and 2. If we eat carbs we need more Vitamin C because the carbs are pushy and won't let the vitamin C get where it needs to go.

You're not going to poop for a month! You need fiber in your diet.

Removing fiber from your diet will shock your system a little. Eating plant based foods requires that our bodies use fiber to help in digestion and passing waste.

Soluble fiber helps food stay in the digestive tract longer so it has more time to be broken down and absorbed. This is needed because so much of plant based food is not easily digested.

Non-soluble fiber helps aid in the movement of waste through the system and adds bulk to your stool. This is needed because so much of plant based food is not easily digested and creates a high amount of waste material.

Our bodies need time to adapt to a no plant food diet. It's been so used to breaking down all this extra stuff that it will take some time for it adapt to the ease of digesting meat. When this happens you should notice a few things.
1. Your poop will be smaller and come out more easily. Meat is dissolved super easy and much more of it is used by the body, so there is significantly less waste.

2. Your poop won't be as stinky. The waste is cleaner and less toxic so it smells less. It's less messy too.
3. You may not poop as often. Some people on the Carnivore Diet have reported only pooping every 3-4 days.

A few things you can try during this phase or anytime if it happens again.

1. Increase your fat intake a little. No one is 100% sure why this helps but it does for some people.
2. Eat more salt. Salt is vital for adrenal and thyroid hormone function which plays big a part in the way our bodies digest and manage food in the body. It also helps manage the acid level in the digestive tract.
3. Drink an herbal tea. There are several that you can try to temporarily relieve constipation.

NOTE: Most people on the Carnivore Diet probably don't get enough salt at first. The change from eating processed food greatly reduced the amount of sodium we get from our food. You will probably want to add good quality sea salt to your diet anyway to make sure you're getting enough. The recommended amount of sodium per day is about 3-5 grams for the average person. 4 grams of sodium is about 2 teaspoons of salt.

Constipation is a real thing and it will most likely hit you at some point. It hit me during weeks two and three. It should get better on its own, within a couple of weeks, just be patient.

Obviously if it becomes excessive, do something about it. Try these remedies or go see a doctor and get help.

My Poop story

I didn't notice anything for a few days. Then after about a week everything kind of slowed down. I felt like I had to push hard to get anything to happen and when it did, there wasn't much there.

Like, dang, that was a lot of work for nothing!

A few days of that then the constipation started. I didn't poop for 2 days at a time but still felt bloated and pressure. This lasted for a little over a week and then I had a big ole party in the pot and was free and clear.

I've had cleaner, smaller, more regular, easier poops from then on.

One thing I've noticed is that I can tell, much faster, when I've eaten something that my body doesn't like. I'm immediately messed up for a day or two after.

The way I poop now is a major contributor to my excitement about this diet.

You're going to have a vitamin deficiency!

This is a topic that I found to be very time-consuming and complicated to figure out. There are 30 or so vitamins and minerals the FDA says we need. After many hours looking for all the places we can get, just Vitamin A from, and what we'd need to eat to get the suggested daily amount, I gave up on getting that much detail for this book.

I could not find any specific study or paper that details how we can get all the vitamins and minerals we need from only eating meat products. I did find a lot of blogs and articles where people break down subsets of vitamins and explain how we don't need plant-based food to get them.

There are also numerous accounts of people on the Carnivore Diet for years who have had no ill side effects due to lack of vitamin intake.

Two suggestions I've seen to help ensure you have enough of the good stuff:

1. Make sure to eat organ meat on some regular basis. Liver in particular is the most nutrient dense meat. I've seen some people say to eat it once a year to once a week. The only real way to know is to get blood tests regularly and adjust as needed.
2. Drink bone broth regularly, this will give you a good boost of collagen and protein and a host of other compounds and minerals that are beneficial to the body.

The question about whether we get enough vitamins from eating only animal products is one of the reasons I emphasize eating high quality meats. Organic, grass fed, pasture raised, etc… is the best way to ensure that you are eating meat that has the nutrients in it you want.

CONSIDERATION: *As I was looking into this topic, the thought occurred to me, "What if there were more things the FDA has in their Recommended Daily Allowance matrix that was wrong because it's based on a mixed diet?" We've just learned that we don't need Vitamin C or Fiber if we're only eating meat. What other vitamins could we leave out and still be healthy?*

Your Gut is going to be ruined. You're going to be sick all the time.

The GUT. What exactly is it?

"The gastrointestinal system, also referred to as the gastrointestinal tract, digestive system, digestive tract, or gut, is a group of organs that includes the mouth, esophagus, stomach, pancreas, liver, gallbladder, small intestine, colon, and rectum. The gut serves many essential roles in sustaining and protecting the overall health and wellness of our bodies, starting with the intake and absorption of nutrients and water." (ref. 3)

Why is this important?
In our guts live a gazillion microbes and bacteria (good and bad) that impact almost everything in our body. The gut is basically a living space for all these bacteria. This is what we call the "Gut Biome". Within the Gut Biome, what we eat has an effect on the balance of good and bad bacteria and how healthy they are.

"The microbiome can be confusing because it's different than other organs in that it's not just located in one location and is not very large in size, plus it has very far-reaching roles that are tied to so many different bodily functions. Even the word "microbiome" tells you a lot about how it works and the importance of its roles, since "micro" means small and "biome" means a habitat of living things.

It's been said by some researchers that up to 90 percent of all diseases can be traced in some way back to the gut and health of the microbiome. Believe it or not, your microbiome is home to trillions of microbes, diverse organisms that help govern nearly every function of the human body in some way. The importance of our gut microbiome cannot be overstated: Poor gut health can contribute to leaky gut syndrome and autoimmune diseases and disorders like arthritis, dementia, heart disease, and cancer, while our health, fertility and longevity are also highly reliant on the balance of critters living within our guts." (ref. 4)

Conventional wisdom says that in order to maintain a healthy gut you need to eat a wide variety of food, animal and plant based. The variety of food we eat is supposed to provide us with things called Prebiotics and Probiotics.

Prebiotics and Probiotics
Prebiotics are substances that encourage the growth of the microbes and bacteria in our gut.

Fiber is probably the most common prebiotic. Outside of our previous fiber discussion, this is a big reason people think you need fiber in your diet.

What many people don't know is that meat has prebiotics, and a good amount of it too.

Prebiotics found in meat:
- Chondroitin
- Casein
- Collagen
- Glucosamine
- Cellulose

So eating meat and animal products can potentially give you all the prebiotics that you need…. Without adding fiber to your diet.

Probiotics are live cultures of microbes and bacteria that are not found in food naturally. Probiotics are added to the Gut Biome to help improve digestion, increase immune function, and help reduce inflammation.

The best source of probiotics is fermented foods. Outside of that, supplements are a common option.

When it comes to the Carnivore Diet, the theory is that with a steady supply of prebiotics in the diet there shouldn't be a need to supplement by adding probiotics.

NOTE: *Gut Biomes differ by person and region, there is not enough data yet to clearly define what a "healthy" Gut Biome looks like.*

Too much protein will kill you.

Have you ever heard of "Rabbit Starvation"? I hadn't until about a month after I started on the Carnivore Diet.

"Protein poisoning was first noted as a consequence of eating rabbit meat exclusively, hence the term, "rabbit starvation". Rabbit meat is very lean; commercial rabbit meat has 50–100 g dissectable fat per 2 kg (live weight). Based on a carcass yield of 60%, rabbit meat is around 8.3% fat while beef and pork are 32% fat and lamb 28%" (ref. 5)

It is possible to die from not eating enough fat. Good thing this diet is a high fat diet!

On the Carnivore Diet you shouldn't have to worry. Fat is king.

From my personal experience, I found that I could target my usual protein goal of 1 gram per pound of lean mass and get to a daily fat:protein ratio of 6-7:3-4.

Red meat causes cancer

OK, this one is getting a little old. There is no direct link to eating red meat and getting cancer. Regardless of what you may hear on the news, eating bacon is not as bad for you as smoking.

Thank goodness!

Here are some very good references with more detailed information than I can provide on what is wrong with the current information being propagated by the media.

Chris Kresser breaks down the latest World Health Organization report and how messed up it is.

"The association between red meat and cancer is not strong (i.e. comparing bacon to cigarettes is absurd), and in fact is often not distinguishable from chance." (ref. 6)

https://chriskresser.com/red-meat-cancer-again-will-it-ever-stop/

Mark Sisson breaks it down a little more and puts it into context with real life.

"There's also the fact that red meat suffers from an "unhealthy user bias." Most heavy red meat eaters aren't sprinting, lifting weights, and going for walks every day.

They're eating their meat between buns, and with fries. They're getting their red meat from Burger King or the 7-11. They can try to control for most of these associations, but it's impossible to account for everything." (ref. 7)

https://www.marksdailyapple.com/what-does-the-who-report-mean-for-your-meat-eating-habit/

In this video, Nina Teicholz walks you through the report and talks about the science behind the "findings' compared to facts.

https://www.youtube.com/watch?v=1rz-8H_i1wA (ref. 8)

There are some relationships that have been identified that have to do with the quality of the meat, its source, and how it's cooked.

Rules of thumb:
- Processed meats are less healthy than plain old meat. (Duh?)
- Grass fed, pasture raised meats are better than grain fed, pen raised meats. (No surprise there.)
- The less you cook the meat the better. Most importantly, burnt meat may increase your risk.

Generally, there is no proof that I can find that red meat causes cancer. I personally will enjoy my daily steak, hamburger, and bacon without worrying about it.

Chapter 4 - What are the benefits of eating nothing but animal parts?

Now that we've addressed some potential risks associated with the Carnivore Diet, let's talk about all the good things that can happen while you're on it.

If you hang around long enough you'll hear some amazing things that Carnivore Diet has done for people. I'm going to break the benefits of being on this diet into 3 main categories.
1. Benefits of eating zero carbs
2. More about fat
3. Anecdotal evidence (that makes sense)

There is a lot of ground to cover learning about the benefits of the Carnivore Diet. People have reported all sorts of amazing results to include healing of IBS, autoimmune diseases, and joint pain. For now this data is anecdotal and has not been studied enough to prove the diet is the mitigating factor in these stories.

This doesn't diminish the value and the weight that these reports have. There are a lot of them, and they all seem to have a surprising level of consistency. For a long list of testimonials from people on what the Carnivore Diet has done for them, go to http://meatheals.com/

Benefits of eating zero carbs

The fat burn

You may not know this but fat is good. Did you know that there is almost no limit to the amount of fat a human can store in their body. It takes less energy to burn fat so it causes less inflammation in the body.

We all know that basically whatever we eat and don't burn off will eventually turn to fat on our bodies. So how does eating fat but not carbs make us burn fat?

Oxidative Priority

Fuel	Alcohol	Ketones	Protein	Carbs	Body Fat
Priority	1	2	3	4	5
Storage	None	Blood	Tissue	Blood	Body
Capacity In Cals	0	20	360-480	1200-2000	Unlimited
Thermic Effect	15%	?	20-35%	5-15%	0-5%

(ref. 9 and 14)

This is the Oxidative Priority chart. It shows how our bodies prioritize and manage the different fuels we use.

Notice that alcohol takes precedence. No matter what's happening, if you put alcohol in, it will burn off first. This is why alcohol is bad for people trying to lose body fat. Drinking stops your body from burning everything else.

See how Carbs have a higher priority than Body Fat? The same thing happens here. The more carbs you have in your system, the less opportunity you have to burn body fat.

Also, notice the Thermic Effect of Carbs vs. Fat. This shows how much energy it takes the body to convert each into usable fuel. This is a % of the total calories available.

If you eat 200 calories of Carbs, then it will take 5-15% of those calories to process what you just ate. You get less available to provide fuel to your body. This means you need to eat more to make up the difference.

This is part of the vicious cycle many people are stuck in.

NOTE: Without getting too complicated, protein is higher in priority but the body uses it to build muscle as its primary function not for fuel. Protein can be used for fuel if the demand is high enough and there isn't enough other fuel sources available.

When we eat carbs our body converts the carbs to glycogen and uses it first. Any leftover carbs get added to the glycogen stores in our muscles and liver. Whatever is left after that goes to our fat stores. Any fat we eat never gets touched and goes right to our fat stores. See where this is going?

As long as we continue to replenish our glycogen stores with more carbs, we never really get a chance to let our bodies burn the fat while the glycogen is in the system

Burning fat off your hips means you have to deplete your glycogen stores enough that your body has to start using fat for fuel more and more as the default. Anytime you put carbs back into the system, you short circuit that process and stop burning fat.

The more used to burning fat your body becomes the more efficient it will be and that's when you will see a reduction of body fat.

The process of burning fat for fuel is called ketosis, this is the basis for the Ketogenic Diet. The Carnivore Diet is very closely related to the Ketogenic diet. They share many of the same benefits because they are both built on similar principles in carb reduction and fat intake.

Reduce insulin resistance

Insulin resistance is an epidemic in much of the modern world. Processed, plant-based (carbs) foods are easy to make, cheap to produce and easy to consume. It's killing us.

NOTE: If you didn't get this from the previous section, Carbohydrates turn into sugars in our system. Glycogen is sugar.

Sugar is the biggest culprit when it comes to insulin resistance. When you eat sugar (straight up or as carbs) your body produces insulin to break down the molecules to be used and stored in the body. The more we eat, the more insulin we need.

When we eat too many carbs, which most people do, our bodies can't keep up and the sugar in our blood increases.

This is insulin resistance and it's how diabetes type 2 starts.

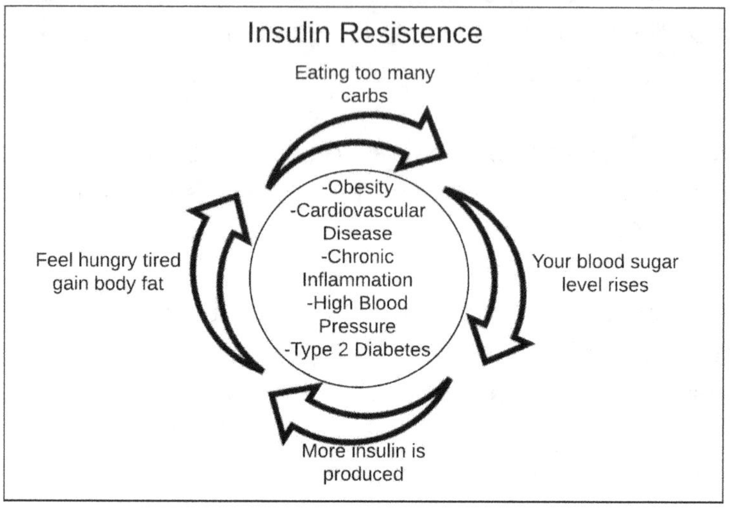

(ref. 10)

Removing carbs from the equation greatly reduces the need for insulin production. This balances out the whole system and improves the symptoms of diabetes and other chronic diseases caused by insulin resistance.

Reduce inflammation

Inflammation is the body's natural reaction to protecting itself from harm. It's a result of the body doing something that is causing it extra stress.

There is a lot of information on how inflammatory some carbohydrates can be. Like much of the information out there you may read completely different interpretations based on the same data.

I'm no scientist, but here's how I view the carbs cause inflammation debate. There is more to the debate than just "carbs are inflammatory". Some carbs may be and some may not be. We have to look at the whole process and ask ourselves what makes sense. Remember, carbohydrates come from plant-based foods. What I've determined from my research tells me that much of the issue lies there.

It takes more energy to process carbs, they have a higher thermic effect than meats.

We get carbs, from plant based foods and it's much more difficult for our systems to digest and process.

If we're eating plant based foods, we need additional nutrients and compounds in our system to handle the extra work our bodies have to perform.

We've determined that our bodies need additional components and processes to digest and excrete plant-based foods.

The more I look at the big picture, the less I'm interested in plan-based foods and dealing with the baggage that comes with them.

More about Fat

Did you know that 60% of the human brain is made of fat?

Maybe it's no coincidence that the commonly suggested amount of daily dietary fat on the Carnivore Diet is 60%-70% of your food.

Wait a second, we just spent a whole section discussing how to reduce fat....

Yup. Adipose tissue (extra fat stored on the body) is the target of the discussion when we talk about fat loss and overall health, This next topic about fat is way more interesting.

The fats we eat are broken down into what's called Fatty Acids. These are used to fuel and support numerous systems in the body.

We are learning more and more about how important a role these fatty acids play in our bodily functions. Take a look at this list of areas in our body that fatty acids have been shown to be an important factor.

In each of these areas there was a noted deficiency of fatty acids, or fatty acids were introduced with some kind of effect to the result.

I took this list from the Oregon State University, Linus Pauling Institute, Micronutrient Information Center information on Essential Fatty Acids. It's a very extensive resource and opened my eyes to how important fats are in our lives. (ref. 11)

- Cell Membrane structure and function
- Vision
- Nervous system
- Regulation of gene expression
- Gestation and Pregnancy
- Coronary Disease
- Stroke
- Alzheimer's
- Diabetes

- Rheumatoid arthritis
- Inflammatory bowel disease
- Asthma
- Major depression and
- Bipolar disorder
- Schizophrenia
- Dementia

There are two main types of dietary fats. This is where we get all the fat we need to make Fatty Acids.
- Saturated
- Unsaturated (Poly and Mono)

Most people know that Unsaturated fats are "good" for us. Did you know that Saturated fats are too? A lot of the benefits we get from fats come from Saturated fats. Good thing there's a healthy amount of it in the animals we eat. (ref. 12)

We can get Saturated AND Unsaturated Fats from fatty beef, lamb, pork, poultry with skin, beef fat (tallow), lard, cream, butter, and cheese. (ref. 13)

Fat is a big part of our lives and I hope you can see one of the reasons it's such a big part of the Carnivore Diet.

Anecdotal Evidence

As if the previous topics weren't enough to give you confidence in your decision to give this diet a try, listen to these claims.

Less need to eat as often

Things we now know 1. Fat is more filling than plant food. 2. Meat is more nutrient dense than plant food. 3. Meat uses less energy to digest than plant food. Is it any surprise that you can feel satisfied for longer after eating just meat, than other foods?

Many people on the Carnivore Diet eat 2 meals a day, that's it. You may be a 1 meal a day person on this diet or a 4 meal a day person. I can tell you that the amount of time you spend thinking about your next meal will be dramatically less.

Easier food prep and lifestyle
This is simple. All you have to do is cook meat.

Sure it can be awkward the first time you go out and order a burger "without a bun, no lettuce, no tomato, no onions, and hold the side of fries, and add a side of bacon", but you get used to it.

Improved fitness and strength
There are stories of strength and performance increases on this diet.

Personally, I have seen an improvement in my recovery and I feel better during a workout than I used to. I have hit personal records since being on the diet. Even after a lower volume of work for a few months while dealing with an injury. Also, my healing improved dramatically after I started this diet.

Easier pooping
Soooo much easier! Less mass in your stool. No smell, no mess, no fuss. Your body uses a much higher percentage of animal based foods and the amount of waste is significantly less.

Once your body gets used to the diet, your poop will become a breeze. You also may not go as much. Some people have said they only go a couple times a week.

No body odor
I have not fully experienced this but the claim is with less inflammation and toxic plant food in our systems, we won't have as much or any body odor. I've seen people that said they no longer use deodorant because they don't need it anymore.

Reduce joint pain
You'll find a lot of stories about people how have relieved arthritis and other joint pain issues. This makes sense to me as meat has many components (collagen, chondroitin, glucosamine etc.) that heal and support joint, and cartilage health.

No sunburns
Really, I'm serious. There is a belief that eating only meat can make sunscreen obsolete. In fact people are saying that sunscreen is the cause of skin cancer, not the sun.

The belief is that the high levels of collagen consumption along with the abundant antioxidants in meat can help the body protect itself from getting burnt.

Disease correction
We touched on this in the section "More about fat". There are many diseases and chronic health issues that people have that are directly related to the consumption of carbs and plant based foods.

Removing those items from a person's diet can have a profound impact on their health.

There's probably more...

I'm sure the longer I study CD and the more feedback I get from people like you, I'll have several things to add to this list.

For now, I hope this gives you an idea of the generally good things that could happen for you on this diet.

Chapter 5 - The first step

My number one goal for you is to stay on this diet as long as possible to see the results you want to see. This chapter is all about getting you started the right way. I don't want you jumping into it blind and not ready to handle the new and wonderful things that are going to happen.

Follow these steps and you'll have a super high chance of getting through 45 days of the diet and seeing amazing results.

Now you're ready to get started, let's go!

What's your "Why"?

Why do you want to do the Carnivore Diet?

When you're at the movies and the smell of popcorn and sight if people eating french fries and candy is all around you, your reason for staying true to your goals must be larger than the surrounding temptations.

This is not a simple, one sentence answer. This should be a very personal picture of what your life could look like if you accomplish what you think this diet can help you accomplish.

If you woke up tomorrow and the Carnivore Diet did everything you hope for, what does that look like to you? How do you feel? What do you do?

That is your "Why".

Set a goal

Figure out why you want to do this diet and write down the results you're looking for.

"I want to lose weight.", doesn't cut it either.

Be S.M.A.R.T

To make sure your goals are clear and reachable, each one should be:

- **S**pecific (simple, sensible, significant).
- **M**easurable (meaningful, motivating).
- **A**chievable (agreed, attainable).
- **R**elevant (reasonable, realistic and resourced, results-based).
- **T**ime bound (time-based, time limited, time/cost limited, timely, time-sensitive).

Specific

Your goal should be clear and specific, otherwise you won't be able to focus your efforts or feel truly motivated to achieve it. When drafting your goal, try to answer the five "W" questions:

- What do I want to accomplish?
- Why is this goal important?
- Who is involved?
- Which resources or limits are involved?

Example: *I want to lose body fat.*

Measurable

It's important to have measurable goals, so that you can track your progress and stay motivated. Assessing progress helps you to stay focused, meet your deadlines, and feel the excitement of getting closer to achieving your goal. A measurable goal should address questions such as:

- How much?
- How many?
- How will I know when it is accomplished?

Example: *I want to lose 5% body fat.*

Achievable

Your goal also needs to be realistic and attainable to be successful. In other words, it should stretch your abilities but still remain possible. When you set an achievable goal, you may be able to identify previously overlooked opportunities or resources that can bring you closer to it. An achievable goal will usually answer questions such as:

- How can I accomplish this goal?
- How realistic is the goal, based on other constraints, such as financial factors?

Example: *I want to lose 5% body fat by eating only meat.*

Tip: Make sure you are setting goals for yourself. Don't be persuaded into saying you want to accomplish something just to make someone else happy, or fulfill what you think someone else's desire for you is. This is your journey, find out what makes you excited about your new life and go that direction.

Relevant

This step is about ensuring that your goal matters to you, and that it also aligns with other relevant goals. We all need support and assistance in achieving our goals, but it's important to retain control over them. So, make sure that your plans drive everyone forward, but that you're still responsible for achieving your own goal. A relevant goal can answer "yes" to these questions:

- Does this seem worthwhile?
- Will this goal have a positive impact on my life?
- Does this match other efforts/needs?

Example: *I want to lose 5% body fat by eating only meat. This will allow me to have more energy to play with my kids.*

Time-bound

Every goal needs a target date, so that you have a deadline to focus on and something to work toward. This part of the SMART goal criteria helps to prevent everyday tasks from taking priority over your longer-term goals. A time-bound goal will usually answer these questions:

- When?
- What can I do six months from now?
- What can I do six weeks from now?
- What can I do today?

Example: *I want to lose 5% body fat, in 45 days, by eating only meat. This will allow me to have more energy to play with my kids.*

My why and my goals

I wanted to do this diet because I wasn't seeing progress in my appearance doing what I was doing. I wasn't happy with how I looked. I was also tired of feeling run down and beat up from my workouts all the time. I had some issues with eating a lot of the foods my wife was making for me. I was tired of being tired. I needed something different.

My goal when I started was just to go 30 days as strict as I could. I hadn't thought it through that much. After the first 2 weeks when I saw 7 pounds gone and over 2% body fat gone, I quickly set some hard goals.

I wanted to get to 10% body fat in 90 days
I wanted to get over some nagging injuries I've been dealing with for months
I wanted to improve all my major workout benchmarks in 90 days

Come up with a plan

Having a plan is the key to knowing when and how to do the things that will get you to your goal.

Your plan will answer questions like these:

- What to eat
- How much to eat
- How to handle exercise
- What to do if you get off your plan

A good plan will take you step by step through the process and help you know what to expect at each phase along the way. This is what we want you to get out of The Meat Life 6-Week Nutrition Plan.

Get people in your camp

Chances are you're going to need some support while you learn how to make these changes. It won't always be fun and with someone to help you along the way, it will make things a lot easier.

My suggestion is to find someone to do it with you. It's nice to have someone you can learn, be challenged, and progress with.

I would also make contact with someone that's done CD for a long enough time to be of help. You can find groups of experienced Zero Carb'ers and Carnivores to ask questions.

NOTE: This feedback may often come in the form of biased opinion. Try to filter out the noise, do a little research on what people are suggesting before you just go do anything.

You might want to get your doctor involved and get your blood drawn for a blood test to set a baseline for your cholesterol and other nutrients. Ya, do that.

If you have access to (or hire one) a certified and licensed nutritionist. They can help guide your intake, meal planning, and generally keep you on track, while making sure you don't short yourself something important along the way.

They may want you to do a body composition test (InBody, Bod Pod, DEXA). I highly recommend doing that. The impact this diet can have on your life is profound and having the numbers to show how major the changes are, is very impactful.

Friends are important. They may not really understand why you're doing this diet. Ask them to be supportive anyway. It can be a lot easier having people around you that won't make jabs at your food choices or eat french fries in front of you.

This is your launching platform

If you do these things and stick with the plan for all 45 days, you will see amazing things start to happen to your body, mind, and soul.

Chapter 6 - The Meat Life Beginner's Guide to the Carnivore Diet

My Method

By the way, I didn't do any of this. I got excited, stopped eating veggies, and just ate whatever I could find in the house that looked like meat. Partially because I couldn't find a book like this and because I can be impulsive, I just jumped in and probably wasted 2 weeks eating bad versions of everything and I came to find out, not eating enough.

After 2 weeks and almost 8 pounds lost, that's a lot in 2 weeks, I figured out that I had been eating an average 300 calorie deficit every day. That's not really a good way to go about this kind of change.

I refocused in my third week and started coming up with the information and planning that I'm reviewing here. I had much more consistent results and, when I made changes, I was able to account for the difference I saw and felt in myself. I hope it helps.

45 Days of Meat

I've seen stories of people who just jumped into this diet and went for broke. Some of them have lasted longer than others but all of them struggled at first. I want you to commit to no less than 45 days of working hard to make this work for you.

Follow the guidelines we've already talked about and start small. Build habits and keep track of the results along the way.

Your plan should be to get your habits in place, help your body adjust, and make some tweaks to get the most out of the diet.

I'm suggesting 45 days because that's how long it took me to get into my groove. The first couple of weeks is going to be mostly adjustment, followed by making small changes. After 3-4 weeks, you should have a good handle on what you need to do to make it a long time on this diet.

Let's Go!

Did you read the last chapter? Do you have a goal in mind?

Awesome, let's get started.

What follows is my guide to help you figure out how to get started and what the Carnivore Diet can do for you.

This is a GUIDE, not a rule book. Use your better judgment and if something is working, keep going. If it's not, then change something to make it better.

Expectations

Change is not easy. Here are some things you may have to deal with as you adapt to this new way of eating.

Reminder: If you go off script during any part of the diet, you may trigger a reversal of your initial adaptation and have to go through these things again.

Constipation

Your body is gonna take a little while, 2-3 weeks on average, to get used to how cleanly you process your food now. Your poop will become less in volume and frequency once you've adapted.

A few things you can try during this phase
1. Increase your fat intake a little. No one is 100% sure why this helps but it does for some people.
2. Eat more salt. Salt is vital for adrenal and thyroid hormone function which plays big a part in the way our bodies digest and manage food in the body. It also helps manage the acid level in the digestive tract.
3. Drink an herbal tea. There are several that you can try to temporarily relieve constipation.

Keto Flu

What is the Keto Flu? It's the time of transition, when your body is adapting from burning carbs for fuel to burning fat for fuel.

There is also a very real addiction component to carbs. In many ways your body is going through sugar withdrawal. Sugar's effect on the body can be just as powerful as cocaine.

These issues can show up in different ways. Commonly reported symptoms of the Keto Flu are:

- Stomach aches or pains
- Brain fog
- Dizziness or confusion
- Nausea
- Irritability
- Diarrhea or constipation
- Muscle cramping or soreness
- Lack of concentration or focus
- Trouble falling or staying asleep
- Sugar cravings
- Heart palpitations

For most people these go away after a week or so. Here are a few things you can do to help get through the Keto Flu.

1. Drink water. It is very important to stay hydrated at all times but with the change your body if going through proper cell hydration is super important to maintain. A good starting place is at least half your body weight in ounces of water each day.

2. Increase your salt intake. This will help with staying hydrated and provide minerals to help your body function.
3. Drink bone broth it provides electrolytes like sodium and potassium while also being hydrating.
4. Increase the fats in your diet. One of the mistakes people make on this diet is cutting out carbs but not replacing it with any fats. This is a primarily fat diet, eat more fat.

Most importantly, give it some time. Unless something really weird is going on or you have another medical issue that is contributing, you should be fine in a week or so.

How much do you need to eat?

This is a subject of much misinformation. The common mantra you'll hear from many people on the Carnivore Diet is "eat when you're hungry and eat until your satiated." The concept is that your body will self-regulate and there is no need to count calories, track macros, or in general do any of that artificial stuff humans do to control their body composition.

In many cases I agree with this concept. It has one major flaw though. It assumes that people are following this diet only for general health purposes. This way of approaching your intake is good if you are OK with letting your body find its own balance over time.

If you have specific goals around fat loss, performance, aesthetics, or anything else, you may need to keep an eye on and track things a little more than that.

Regardless of what you think is the best way to make the diet work, for these first 6 weeks I think it's good to track a few things as far what you're putting into your mouth. This is a guideline that I follow and I use it as a base for any changes I want to make. Not because the numbers themselves matter, but because the data they provide lets me know how far I can go, or shouldn't go as I make changes to my intake.

I HIGHLY recommend tracking your daily protein intake in grams, and keeping an eye on how much fat you're eating as a percentage of your daily intake.

A good rule of thumb is to eat 1 x your lean mass weight in grams of protein and to keep fat to around 60% - 70% of your total daily intake. This is a good starting point. You can plan meals around this. You can shop and have an idea of how much food you need for a week. If it doesn't meet your needs after a couple weeks, then increase or decrease the fat % or protein grams. Experiment with it. Find out what works for you.

No one can tell you how much you need to eat. This is a simple diet to follow and the changes that you may need to make are simple too. If you aren't seeing the results you're looking for then play around with the numbers until you get something that works.

You have to take some level of owner here. You can't just ask the Internet what you should do. Sometimes it takes a little trial and error.

If you aren't keeping track of what you've tried then you'll waste time making the same mistakes over and over. Even if you don't track things forever, humor me and do it for these 6 weeks. You might learn something.

Yes, you don't NEED to track anything. I think it's a little irresponsible to yourself not to.

Making Changes

So you're only going to eat meat and animal products for 6 weeks. What do you eat? What don't you eat? How much do you eat?

Since this is what's happening starting day one, let's answer come of the most common questions. We'll also discuss what you can get rid of in the beginning.

Your first week is your baseline week. Everything you do from here is an adjustment off the initial changes you make.

What to eat

We talked about it a little already but there are a few different categories of things to eat.

- Meat
- Dairy
- By-Products
- Beverages

Meat

Here is what Dr. Mabry has to say about his eating habits in the same interview we pulled from earlier.
https://zerocarbzen.com/2016/05/24/zero-carb-interview-dr-paul-mabry-m-d/

"I rarely eat steak, usually only at restaurants when I'm traveling or eating out with friends, but when I do, I prefer it rare. I buy 3 lb chubs of 27% fat hamburger from my local Kroger which fortunately for me regularly puts them on sale for $5.99 to draw customers. I go every day that week and get my 2 allowed chubs and freeze them. I make a casserole with 2 lbs of hamburger mixed with 8 beaten eggs and laid in a casserole dish liberally slathered with butter then I cover it with 4 cups (about 1 lb) of grated Aged Cheddar cheese which I regularly get from Kroger in 2 lb blocks for $7.49 sometimes on sale for $6.49 (I stock up and freeze). I bake this at 325 for 30 minutes and cut into 6 squares. I eat 1 square every day for lunch. For those of you who are interested, this gives me 21 grams of protein in the hamburger, 9 grams of protein in the eggs and 18 grams of protein in the cheese for a total of 48 grams of protein at lunch.

For dinner, I almost always eat about 10 ounces of a combination of all beef sausage and hotdogs. Both contain Offal which is "organ meat" which is higher in vitamins and minerals than steak, plus I eat another 3 ounces of Aged Cheddar Cheese. There are 40 grams of protein in the sausage and hot dogs and 21 grams in the cheese for a total of 61 grams of protein in the evening meal and 109 grams of protein for the day. Which is less than 1.5 kg of protein per kg of ideal body weight for me."

For most people eating this way, the fatter the cut of meat the better. A majority of people like to eat ribeye steak as it is one of the fattest cuts. 6 of the fattiest cuts of meat that I've found are:

- NY Strip Steak (34 grams of fat in a 7 oz. cut)
- Ribeye Steak (54 grams of fat in an 11 oz. cut)
- Delmonico Steak (50 grams of fat in an 8 oz. cut)
- Skirt Steak (30 grams of fat in a 9 oz. cut)
- Pork Ribs (26 grams of fat in an 8 oz. cut)
- Chicken Thighs (34 grams of fat in an 8 oz. cut)

There are so many options for what kind of meat you could eat. I could write a book just on that but that would be too much work.

Just keep in mind that it's important to have an idea of the fat % in the cuts of meat you eat. In general, chicken, fish, and pork are leaner and may need added fats like butter when you cook them.

Cooking meat
How much you cook the meat can affect the nutrients and properties of the meat. There are some people who follow a raw meat diet because they want the most out of the meat they can get. (Not me).

I suggest that there be some pink to red showing in the meat when you eat it. If you've never heard of reverse searing, go look it up. It makes for a really good steak.

Seasoning

Keep it simple. For most of what I cook, I use salt and pepper. Seeing as how I live near Baltimore, MD I have an abundant supply of Old Bay Seasoning available and I use it frequently as well.

Don't use anything with sugar or additives. Here are some suggestions for companies that make spices that would work:

- Redmon https://redmond.life
- Balanced Bites https://bbspices.com/
- Primal Palate
  https://www.primalpalate.com/organic-spices/

If you want to put a garlic clove on your steak, then put a dang garlic clove on your steak. My suggestion though, wait until after the 45 days when your body is more settled into your new way of eating. If you want the flavors of whole herbs, cook with them then leave them to the side.

Note: The only condiment I use is mustard or hot pepper sauce. I have learned to like it a lot.

Processed Meats

This is where I got stuck the first two weeks I started. I didn't make a plan, so I just ate whatever I had at home or could find when I went out. It's all just meat right?? Wrong.

- Hotdogs
- Sausage
- Jerky
- Bratwurst
- Deli meat

These are easy to get and easy to eat. That means they probably aren't as good for you. Processed meats have added chemicals and THEY'RE PROCESSED. Have you ever looked at the ingredient labels on this stuff? Do it.

I'm not suggesting to never eat them although that probably would be for the best.

You can find better versions, but they aren't as readily available, and they can be more expensive. If you're going to get these meats, find a local butcher that makes their own, find out what goes into them, and have fun.

Organ Meat

This is the good stuff. It's also some of the hardest to eat for most people. It can be smelly, gamey, and not easy to eat. It's also the most nutrient packed food there is.

Of course there is nothing saying that you HAVE to eat organ meat. Some people on the Carnivore Diet, don't eat any. Personally I think it's a wise choice to include organ meat on some regular basis. I'm not convinced that I'm just as good without it. I mean, when you watch a lion eating a gazelle it always goes right for the guts doesn't it? There has to be something there we can learn from. ;-)

Take a look at Beef Liver. It's amazing. My goal is to include at least 1 serving of liver into my meals 1-2 times in a two-week period.

I'm not a super fan of it fried. Instead, my wife makes a good pate that I mix with some cream cheese and dip pork rinds in. It's actually kind of good that way.

Dairy

I eat about 2-4 slices of cheese a week. (I'm considering cutting this out though) I have 1-2 tbsp of butter every morning in my coffee. I also cook my eggs, and some steaks in butter.

I love it.

In my definition of the Carnivore Diet, the only real requirement is that what I eat should have been alive or part of something that was alive at one point. Dairy fits the bill.

If you decide to include dairy, make sure it's as whole and natural as you can get. Full fat is the way to go.

Couple of things to remember though. You will have to test this stuff out.

Many people are lactose intolerant or allergic. This can show up in a handful of different ways.

- Skin conditions
- IBS
- Excess mucus
- Joint Inflammation

Dairy contains sugars which cause an insulin response and may contribute to you not losing the fat you are trying to lose. Try a week with it and a week without it. See what happens.

Animal By-Products

This is the "other stuff" things that we eat. Here's a short list of things I consider to be OK on the Carnivore Diet even though it's not just meat:

- Pork Rinds
- Bone Broth
- Bone Marrow
- Ghee
- Eggs

I say go for it. As with any of the food you eat, look for no added anything, no sugar, and stay away from stuff you know is crap.

Beverages

What can you drink on this diet?

Water.

Seriously, that's it. Learn to love water. Honestly, since I've been doing this, I have appreciated water a lot more. When I do get thirsty, I'm really thirsty, and it tastes so good.

If you need a little something more, get some lightly flavored carbonated water. La Croix's, Refresh, or something similar. Stuff with no added sugar or sweeteners, just some carbonation and a little flavor.

The Exception

If you're like me, you need your coffee. I have one every morning. I won't say more about this than, if you want one go for it.

My suggestion, whatever you do, do it consistently for the 45 days. I would only stop if you've stalled, tried everything else, and drinking coffee is the last thing you have to change.

What not to eat

How simple is this? …. If it's not in the "What to eat" section, don't eat it.

No plant-based food
Nothing that comes in a box
Nothing that has an ingredient label
Nothing with sauces or bastes
Nothing with added anything
No nuts or beans
No bread or breading
No veggies

Supplements

There are only three things I take outside of what I get in my food. I've actually been supplementing with these for several years. I highly recommend that you take these as well.

- Magnesium
- Fish Oil
- Vitamin D

Magnesium is lacking in most people's diet. There are some theories as to why, but it's best to just supplement.

Fish oil and Vitamin D can be ingested based on what you eat. If you aren't eating a lot of fatty fish, then I would supplement.

Here is the best stuff I can suggest for you to get. https://www.puori.com

I have not seen a need to take anything else. If you want to take a multivitamin for your own sense of well-being then go for it.

For sports performance I just keep eating meat. Meat has all the components for building muscle. There shouldn't be a need for Creatine, and definitely not a need for BCAA's (branch chain amino acids).

Putting it all together

Now that we have all the do's and don'ts out of the way, how do we come up with what to eat every day?

I'm going to go through my process. I'll walk you through it and hopefully you can use it to make your own plan.

PREP STEP: Go get an InBody body composition scan or a DEXA scan, or something that will give you:

- Body weight
- Lean Mass
- Skeletal Muscle Mass
- Base Metabolic Rate
- Body Fat %

Step 1 - Setting my goals

This could be a long list of things. Everyone is going to have a different set of goals for this diet. In most cases we can boil them down to some general categories.

Weight/Fat Loss - This goal is all about reducing the amount of body fat you have. There may be some muscle gain and other benefits, but really you just want to drop the excess.

Weight/Strength Gain - If getting stronger is your goal then you're going to have to eat a little more and your workouts will play a big role in how you progress.

General Health Improvement - There a many people who are using the Carnivore Diet to heal their bodies. They may not specifically have a weight goal. Some people have skin conditions, IBS, autoimmune disease, or any of a number of other issues. The Carnivore diet has shown to improve a lot of these conditions. This is more of a maintenance goal with the cleaner intake of food being the target.

Something to think about

This diet is zero carb. Every goal you have is going to result in some sort of fat loss as a foundation. Isn't that cool! Regardless of what goal you choose, there are only a few things you have to keep in mind.

1. How much protein do you need?
2. How much fat do you need?
3. Are your meat choices varied enough?
4. How do you feel?

Your protein intake will vary based on your goal (up, down, or maintain). Your fat intake may need to change based on how you feel and it should match your protein intake by %. Make sure you eat different meats to get all the benefits they have to offer (Steak is still the base). Your body will tell you if something isn't right. Pay attention.

My goals

1. 10% Body Fat in 90 days. I started at 16.7%
2. I want to maintain my current Skeletal Muscle Mass. I started at 93.9 lbs.
3. I want to keep my athletic performance at the same level or improve.

My primary goal falls into the Lose Fat category.

Regardless of your goal. I think everyone should start with a goal of eating 1 x their lean mass weight in grams of protein. Let's see how that works out using my numbers.

Step 2 - How much protein and fat

My numbers when I started were:

- Weight: 197.9 lbs
- Body Fat %: 16.7
- Skeletal Muscle Mass: 93.9 lbs.
- Lean Mass: 164.8 lbs.
- Body Fat Weight: 33.1 lbs.
- Base Metabolic Rate (BMR): 1900 cals

My BMR was 1900 calories per day. We know for a fact that a daily calorie deficit will not only facilitate fat loss but muscle loss as well. I didn't want that.

Looking at my Lean Mass of 164.8 lbs, I want to eat 165 grams of protein each day.

Protein has 4 calories per gram, so I need to eat 660 calories of protein daily. That means I should get about 1240 calories of fat daily as well.

Sounds like a lot, doesn't it? Let's double check the number by looking at percentages.

On the Carnivore Diet I recommend somewhere between 60% and 70% daily fat intake.

Using these numbers I can figure out what % of fat I'll get with that amount of calories.

1240 / 1900 = 65% of the total calories per day.

Bingo! Right where I want it to be.

Adjusting to meet my goals

I didn't go through this process for the first two weeks after I started.

When I got my body composition done at 14 days, I was 8 pounds lighter and 2 pounds of that was muscle. I wasn't eating enough. I had to adjust.

The first thing I did was figure out the numbers we just went over. I had to include one other factor before I could start planning to make my meals.

Working out and exercise

Your activity level affects your overall calorie usage on top of what your BMR is.

Reminder: *BMR is also called the Netflix and Chill number. It is what calories your body burns each day if you literally sat on your butt and did nothing for 24 hours.*

Generally speaking we can use the following table to calculate a number closer to what we realistically burn each day.

Activity Level	Multiply x BMR
Sedentary (Not active much)	x1.2
Light Active (Walking, Yoga)	x1.375
Moderately Active (CrossFit, HIIT)	x1.5
Extremely Active (Competitive Athlete)	x1.75

Taking this into consideration I calculated what my overall calorie goals should be. Keep in mind this is going to change both the protein and fat amounts for each day.

Rest Days

On days that I'm not working out I consider myself to still be fairly active, so I use the Light Active multiplier.

BMR 1900 x 1.375 = 2612 calories

Now I need to know what that converts to in fat and protein.

*2612 * .65 = 1698 cals of fat and 2612 - 1698 = 914 cals of protein*

What does this mean? Well, this is the info I need to know how many grams of food I can eat each day.

Fat has 9 calories per gram. Protein has 4 calories per gram.

On my rest days, I can have 188 grams of fat and 228 grams of protein. We'll get into how much food that is later in this section.

Let's look at my workout days.

Workout Days

I'm a CrossFitter, so I'm going to use the Moderately Active multiplier of 1.5 to figure this out.

BMR 1900 x 1.5 = 2850 calories
*2850 * .65 = 1852 cals of fat and 2850 - 1852 = 998 cals of protein*

Total Grams needed on workout days:
Fat = 205 grams
Protein = 250 grams

Now I know how much food I need to eat each day. Time to go shopping!

Step 3 - Meal Planning

Figuring out what foods to eat and how much of each is the hardest part of the process. Every kind of meat has different percentages and amounts of fat and protein.

You have to put in a little effort to figure out what will work for you. There are plenty of websites you can go to that have nutrition info to let you know the fat and protein content of specific cuts and kinds of meat. Here are a couple:

https://www.myfitnesspal.com

http://nutritiondata.self.com/

This isn't comprehensive but here is a table with general info for the common meats. (info is for uncooked meat)

Meat	Amount	Fat grams	Protein grams	Caloric Fat %
Ribeye Steak	1 Pound	96g	80g	73%
Chicken Thighs	1 Pound	19g	89g	32%
Pork Ribs	1 Pound	50g	92g	55%
Salmon	1 Pound	28.8g	89.6g	42%

You will get better caloric fat percentages out of beef. Many people on the Carnivore Diet only eat steaks.

Scheduling your meals

This can get complicated or you can keep it simple. You're not going to feel as hungry as often with the increased fat intake.

I tried to break my total calories into 4 manageable chunks I felt I could eat in one sitting. This puts me about to 3/4 pounds of meat per meal.

Look at your schedule and do what works best for you. When do you have time? When do you get hungry?

At this point don't worry about intermittent fasting or timing meals with workouts too much. Just plan it out so you never feel like you're hungry.

Example of my day when I workout

Time	Meal	Fat grams	Protein grams
6:00 am	Bulletproof Coffee	26g	
9:00 am	5 Eggs, 5 pieces bacon	105g	95g
12:00pm	¾ Ground Beef	48g	60g
3:00 pm	9 oz Canned Tuna	15g	49g
6:00 pm	.5 lbs Sirloin Steak	8g	50g

This gives me a total of 202 Fat grams and 254 Protein grams, which is right on with my goals

Summary

This is the process you should start with to figure out what works and doesn't. I don't think you'll need to do all this work after 4-6 weeks. Once you figure out what works for you, it's really easy to go with the flow and have a good understanding of where you are each day.

This part is important though. Track your data and LEARN from it. If you don't do this stuff in the beginning, I promise you'll end up spinning your wheels at some point and you won't know what to do.

Fat vs. Protein

One of the things you need to remember is that using your BMR and calories to determine how much fat you need is just the starting point. You may not need that many calories each day depending on your goals and activity level.

There are no hard and fast rules. Everything can be variable.

Keep in mind that fat uses less energy to process and it has more energy by volume than carbs so you don't need as much to get the same amount of energy.

If you have a body fat loss goal then you need to eat even less fat by % because you want your body fat to be the priority for fuel consumption, not the fat you eat. (In general, I'd not recommend going lower than 50%)

Protein will be your base factor, figure the rest from there. If you're losing muscle mass, it's most likely that you're in a protein deficit not a caloric deficit. On the Carnivore Diet you can be in a total caloric deficit by BMR and still add muscle if you're getting enough protein.

Don't worry about tracking ketones, or any of that. If you're not eating carbs, you'll be in ketosis. Use your body composition changes to determine how it's working for you.

What happens after 6 weeks?

During your 6 weeks, you should be trying to find a way to fit your new way of eating into your lifestyle. If you are successful, you may not want to go back to what you did before.

Also, you may really want a pizza.

When I hit 6 weeks, I was even more intent on continuing. If you want to keep going, then here are a few things I suggest.

1. Retest your body composition. You're going to feel different and look different. Get the numbers to show you what actually happened to your body.
2. If you can get a blood test, get one. Get lipid (NMR+Lipid w/LDL-P), Insulin, and Glucose panels.
3. Do more research on recipes, ways to cook meat, and find other people that are having success eating carnivore.

If you don't think this diet is for you, then here's what I suggest.

One thing at a time.

If you really cut everything else out, then only introduce one thing at a time for a few days before you add something else.

If you've cut out milk and cheese, start eating them again for 3 or 4 days. PAY ATTENTION to your body and ask yourself. "Since I've been eating dairy again what has changed about my body and how I feel?"

You could add in leafy greens first, or nuts, or maybe you really miss your zucchini and squash. It doesn't matter

Whatever it is. The best way to find out how your body is reacting to different foods is to go slow. You're starting with a clean slate. Your body is refreshed and will react if it gets something it doesn't like.

Listen to what it's telling you and learn from it.

Stay in touch

Follow us on Instagram at **@the_meatlife**
Like us on Facebook at **@themeatlife**
Follow the Blog at http://themeatlife.com

Helpful Links

Facebook Groups and Pages

@themeatlife - The Meat Life is my page where I post information about the Carnivore Diet, updates on my experience, product reviews, and tips about being a carnivore.

@worldcarnivoretribe - This is a group dedicated to the Carnivore Diet. It's pretty active and you can usually get some good info from it.

@zerocarbdoc - Zero Carb Doc is Dr. Mabry's Facebook group. Very good resource. Dr. Mabry is active in it and always helpful.

@principiacarnivora - This is a really good group to get in. There are a lot of people who have been ZC for a long time-sharing info. It has the largest membership of any group I've found yet.

Websites and Blogs

http://themeatlife.com - This is my blog. Similar to my FB page but I tend to get a little deeper into topics and spend a little more time breaking things down.

https://zerocarbzen.com - This is Esmée La Fleur's blog. So much good info. Go check it out.

http://www.empiri.ca - This site is run by Amber O'Hearn. Amber has helped many people through sharing her own experiences and is partly my inspiration for writing this book.

http://justmeat.co - One of the best sources of links to other resources, studies, and information about the Carnivore Diet.

http://www.zerocarbhealth.com/ - Maybe the oldest and most comprehensive site there is on the Zero Carb lifestyle.

http://meatheals.com/ - Great place to go learn about other people and what this diet has done for them.

References

Reference Number	Reference	Location
1	https://en.wikipedia.org/wiki/Scurvy	Your going to get scurvy
2	https://autoimmunethyroid.wordpress.com/2006/09/04/why-meat-prevents-scurvy/?hc_location=ufi	Your going to get scurvy
3	https://med.nyu.edu/medicine/gastro/about-us/gastroenterology-news-archive/your-gut-feeling-healthier-digestive-system-means-healthier	Your gut is going to be ruined
4	https://draxe.com/microbiome/	Your gut is going to be ruined
5	https://en.wikipedia.org/wiki/Protein_poisoning	Protein Poisoning
6	https://chriskresser.com/red-meat-cancer-again-will-it-ever-stop/	Red meat will give you cancer
7	https://www.marksdailyapple.com/what-does-the-who-report-mean-	Red meat will give you cancer

	for-your-meat-eating-habit/	
8	https://youtu.be/1rz-8H_i1wA	Red meat will give you cancer
9	http://mariamindbodyhealth.com/happens-eat-many-carbohydrates/	Benefits of no carb diet
10	https://www.ditchthecarbs.com/what-is-insulin-resistance/	Benefits of no carb diet
11	http://lpi.oregonstate.edu/mic/other-nutrients/essential-fatty-acids#membrane-structure-function	More about fat
13	https://wellnessmama.com/1265/saturated-fat/	More about fat
12	http://nutritiondata.self.com/	More about fat
14	https://www.bodybuilding.com/fun/ask-the-macro-manager-what-is-thermic-effect.html	More about fat
15	https://www.ncbi.nlm.nih.gov/pubmed/20071648	Scientific Proof
16	https://www.healthline.com/nutrition/saturated-fat-good-or-bad#section3	Scientific Proof

| 17 | https://www.healthline.com/nutrition/5-studies-on-saturated-fat | Scientific Proof |
| 18 | https://www.ncbi.nlm.nih.gov/pmc/articles/PMC2974200/ | Scientific Proof |

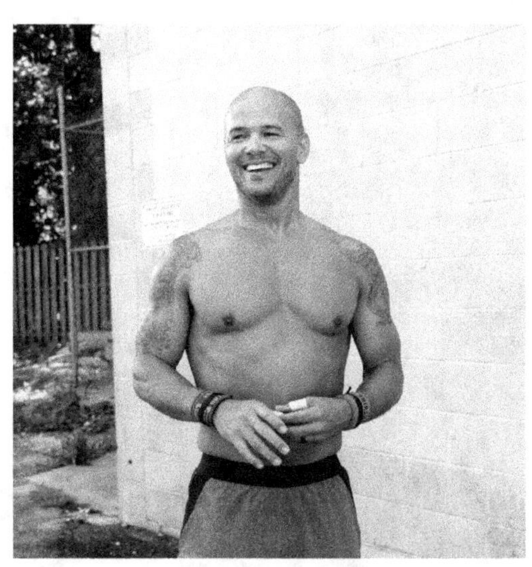

Author: Bronson Dant
bronson@themeatlife.com
*Now: 185 lbs., 12% body fat and feeling great!
I dropped 15 lbs and over 4% body fat in under 2 months,
and I've been able to maintain it.*

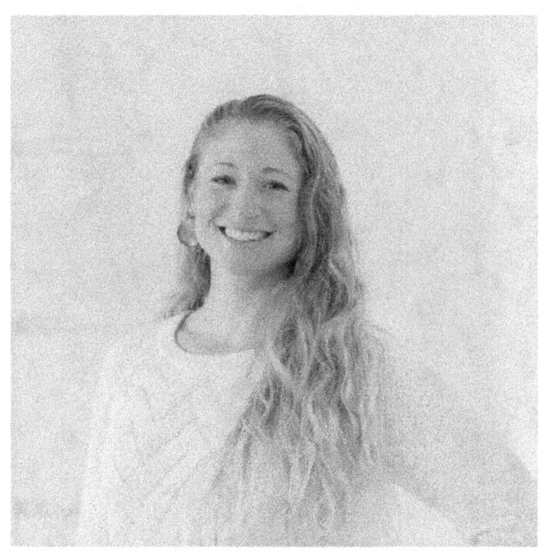

Co-Author: Jamie Dant
http://otbnutrition.net